The Unsupported Middle

future developments in a primary care-led NHS

The Unsupported Middle

future developments in a primary care-led NHS

Geoff Meads

June Huntington

Peter Key

Peter Mumford

Eleanor Brown

Kathryn Evans

Foreword by
Dame Rennie Ritchie

Radcliffe Medical Press
Oxford and New York

© 1997 The authors

Radcliffe Medical Press Ltd
18 Marcham Road, Abingdon, Oxon OX14 1AA, UK

Radcliffe Medical Press, Inc.
141 Fifth Avenue, New York, NY 10010, USA

British Library Cataloguing in Publication Data

A catalogue record for this book is available from the British Library.

ISBN 1 85775 109 4

Library of Congress Cataloging-in-Publication Data is available.

Typeset by Advance Typesetting Ltd, Oxon
Printed and bound by Biddles Ltd, Guildford and King's Lynn

CONTENTS

ABOUT THE AUTHORS

Eleanor Brown is the Practice Development and Fundholding Manager at the Paxton Green Group Practice. For the past 13 years she has worked in both community and primary health care, moving from field work into management. After a short period of planning and development work, she took up her present position in primary health care for a general practice in South London providing an extended range of services to 19 000 people. The practice is a first-wave fundholder and Eleanor heads the project, with two partners as advisers. Paxton Green is one of eight national nurse prescribing sites and is involved in a total purchasing project. She is Chair of the Lambeth Southwark & Lewisham GP Fundholding Forum and an executive member of the National Association of Fundholding Practices. Primary care organizational development and managed health care are particular work interests. Learning to ballroom dance helps to maintain her sense of humour.

Kathryn Evans is a consultant to groups and organizations working with change. She is currently seconded to the London Health Partnership, based at the King's Fund, helping to develop 'whole systems' approaches to improving primary care services for older people living in cities. These approaches involve working across organizational boundaries, putting users at the centre of dialogue and development.

June Huntington PhD is an independent consultant in health care management and a Visiting Fellow of the King's Fund. She has worked with general practice for over 20 years and currently works with organizations at every level of the primary care system. She speaks and writes widely on health policy and its impact on the development of practices and health authorities, and on general practice as a profession. She has published *Managing the Practice: whose business?* (1995) Radcliffe Medical Press, Oxford, and co-authored *The Primary Care Challenge* (1995) Churchill Livingstone, Edinburgh. She has also contributed to Meads G (ed.) (1995) *Future Options for General Practice*, Radcliffe Medical Press, Oxford and Meads G (ed.) (1996) *A Primary Care-led NHS: putting it into practice*, Churchill Livingstone, Edinburgh.

Peter Key is a consultant and Director of Dearden Management, an organizational development consultancy which specializes in health and health care issues. While his consultancy work covers all aspects of organizational development, he has a particular interest in strategy development, performance management and evaluation. Most of his work is with top teams and individual managers responsible for bringing about significant organizational change. In addition to his UK clients, Peter regularly works in Poland and Spain. His career experience includes periods as a navigator in the merchant navy, an operational manager and then Chief Executive in the NHS, and as the first Director of Management Development for the NHS in England and Wales.

Professor Geoff Meads recently joined the City University, Health Management Group from the NHS in the South and West where he was a Regional Director from 1992–96. Prior to this, he was a FHSA Chief Executive. His recent publications include *Future Options for General Practice* (1995) Radcliffe Medical Press, Oxford and *A Primary Care-led NHS: putting it into practice* (1996) Churchill Livingstone, Edinburgh.

Peter Mumford has worked with the King's Fund in London for 12 years. He is a consultant in organization and leadership development with a strong commitment to improving public health services. He works with hospitals, health authorities, local authorities and general practices, senior management groups, boards, clinical teams and individual leaders. He has also designed and directed many programmes for senior managers and clinicians. On three occasions he has been seconded to hospitals undergoing major change, as external facilitator and process consultant – the most recent to the Royal Perth Hospital, Perth, Western Australia.

FOREWORD: TOUCHING TOMORROW

Like most other regions, the South and West was born out of a merger of two earlier regions. It was clear to me, and to many others within this region, that the most desirable national health service of tomorrow would exhibit the benefits of appropriate, valued individual contributions *and* integrated, coherent team-working. It was also abundantly clear that getting key stakeholders together for a simultaneous 360 degree focus, dialogue, analysis and learning would be far more productive than the incremental 'pass-the-parcel' process we so often experience.

Most of those who work for and with the NHS have enough to do coping with the legacy of yesterday and endeavouring to manage today. Yet it is these same people who must translate today's challenges and aspirations into a meaningful tomorrow.

The Unsupported Middle conference was a continuation of an approach we had used in our policy development groups and clinical briefing for boards. It also helped us to practise what we were preaching by mirroring, by its process, what we believe to be an essential way of working.

Ideally, conferences should be about 'conferring'. All too often they are about sitting and listening. This event, like the others in the series, made sure that we all engaged, at many levels, for the duration of the conference and well beyond. There was an enormous amount of enthusiasm to take part and contribute from a wide range of people. From the start, I was keen to give my wholehearted support to this event and this way of working.

I believe that the NHS as an organization should be life-affirming for all those who use the service and all those who work within it. For 'the unsupported middle' to become 'the heart of the matter' we must strive together to make sure we have the 'will to be wholehearted'. For if we drop the 'w' it leaves us 'ill' and 'hole hearted' and we will quickly return to 'the unsupported middle'.

Dame Rennie Ritchie
September 1996

1 The unsupported middle: an introduction

Geoff Meads

They were the last group to report and, according to popular stereotype, the least promising. Largely central appointees and female, the most senior in both status and age, their feedback to the rest of the participants in a regional learning event entitled *The Unsupported Middle*, seemed destined to be the most conservative. Not that it would really matter; the material from the first four groups had been sufficiently stimulating. There was more than enough for the facilitators to exploit over the remaining two days of the programme.

The purchaser chief executives group had mapped the relationships of the reformed NHS on an imaginary dartboard; covered with one-off 'hits'. Around the bull's-eye were stuck three pieces of paper bearing the titles 'Secretary of State', 'GPs' and 'HA chief executives' – of course. This triumvirate of power was surrounded by a bewildering mosaic of other paper patches and concentric circles, the meanings of which were too hard to read, let alone understand, from any distance away. In short, it was chaos theory; the reformed NHS – too complex to communicate, with GPs and Ministers in exclusive control and top level management mediating between them.

The provider representatives were a little less graphic. The 'electrical circuit' they drew rather pathetically contained few points and quickly looped back to the original socket; the NHS Trust itself. The Community Trust did have a 'terminal' with the social services department, but otherwise its circuit followed the same sparse lines as its Acute counterpart. Together they had lost contact with the external NHS. They did not really know what was going on in the wider world.

The primary care team players felt very much the same, at least at practice management level. Their image of the reformed NHS was of a five-layer pyramid with the Government and NHS Executive at the top; providers and purchasers, the solid intervening layers; and general practice, the burgeoning bottom tier. There was only one problem with this expansion – the overall height of the pyramid was not changing. The pressure at the bottom was simply much greater, getting closer and closer to bursting point and those at the top of the pyramid remained out of sight and out of reach.

A galaxy of stars, planets and constellations was the image of the fourth set of stakeholders: service users and their representatives. Shooting stars and short-life meteorites (GP fundholders, health authorities and purchasing strategies) briefly caught the eye but it was the Department of Health as the Sun that dominated the skyline. While the former burnt out, this everlasting orb blazed ever more brightly, shedding light on all those that stayed within its rays. The users and carers were not sure that they should have been paired, but together they knew exactly to whom they should still relate in the reformed NHS.

After four such vivid and varying illustrations of subjective reality in the reformed NHS, it seemed there could be little more to add when, unexpectedly, all those in the non-executive member stakeholder group got up and came to the front of the room. They stood Indian file with one of their number set apart, calling the tune. At her instruction, the leader of the line spoke: 'It is the pre-primary care-led NHS and I am the consultant, and I lead the NHS'.

'And I am a university and I follow the consultant' said the next in line.

'Me too' echoed the third person, an NHS manager.

'And I am a GP and I am where I am used to being – stuck in the middle and unable to get out' said the next, facing the back of the manager, who was facing the back of the university representative ahead of him.

Next in the row was the Community Health Council (CHC) complaining of neglect but still looking, nevertheless, in exactly the same direction as the others; and then finally, after an interval of time and space, came the patient: 'I'm at the back and I cannot even see the front of the queue. That's where the consultant is, isn't it? I thought he was meant to be looking after me'.

The member set apart from the line then spoke again, announcing: 'I am the Regional Chair. It is 1 April 1996. The primary care-led NHS is upon us'.

What happened next? Who moved in the column? Certainly not the consultant who stayed at its head. The university representative remarked that she only changed course 'very slowly' and even the GP was reluctant to shift his stance until sharply reminded again that these were the days of the *Primary care*-led NHS, which left him facing the CHC for the first time – with disturbing effect.

'I don't like this at all' said their representative. 'Now we are faced with all these local practices. There are far too many of them for us to cope with and most of them won't let us in. Even if they do, we cannot see what they are up to. It's not like ward rounds; the consulting room door is always shut'.

One person did make a 180 degree turn – the NHS manager, as directed. But this did not last long. In a parting statement, the RHA Chair proclaimed an eight per cent reduction in 'overheads'. The NHS manager stepped aside and then so too did the RHA Chair herself. They were no longer on the map of the reformed NHS, leaving it as it was before – in the same order only with wider gaps. The patient's concluding cry was the same: 'I am still at the back and now nobody seems to know where we should be going. I liked the sound of a primary care-led NHS, but who now is going to make it happen?'

This account of how relationships are seen in the NHS of the 1990s describes, I hope, the changing and different perceptions of its chief constituents more accurately and powerfully than any organizational diagram or formal description of roles and responsibilities could ever do. Of course, quite properly, NHS communications continue to concentrate on the latter, but it is essential if 'primary care-led' is to be translated from policy into practice, that the map of relationships which explains actual behaviour is understood, so that the balance of power can genuinely be shifted.

It was the conclusion, and conviction, that this shift needs to be made towards those who have in the past been on the periphery of the NHS, that led to the South and West regional learning event entitled *The Unsupported Middle*. The event was the third in a series going under the banner of *The Primary Care Challenge*; the first two parts of which had pinpointed specifically community health services, practice managers and CHCs as 'the unsupported middle'.[1] This phrase, suggesting a lack of belonging, a sense of hollowness and above all the absence of power, captured the imagination of many of those working in the South and West NHS region. At a time when professional, political and managerial languages have fought for ascendancy, its soundbite quality seemed to help. *The Unsupported Middle* captured what many felt and thought, and not just from those in the three categories listed above.

Accordingly, *The Unsupported Middle* as a learning event was planned with some basic assumptions. The informal organization of the NHS has become more significant in its decision-making. At local level, these decisions increasingly owe more to informal participative processes than they do to central planning directives. (Operational dissonance and even subversion occurs in the NHS when too many staff and patients are required to do what they do not believe in.) Understanding the NHS today therefore requires less rational interpretation and more behavioural analysis. Real learning has to be experiential.

In formal terms, the event had five objectives:

1 to explore the power bases and relationships within a primary care-led NHS
2 to examine critically the obstacles and tensions attached to moving to new ways of working
3 to gain a deeper understanding of the behavioural patterns, values and beliefs which now determine NHS processes and relationships
4 to learn more about the different perceptions, problems and aspirations of key stakeholder groups for the NHS
5 to define the new relationships required at individual, group and organizational levels.

These objectives are, perhaps, more easily presented and understood as a simple set of questions:

• Who is in control of the NHS and is it changing?
• Where are we going and who or what is getting in the way?
• Is there still an NHS consensus?
• How do each of us see a primary care-led NHS and what do we want out of it?
• How should we relate to each other now?

The nature of such questions is fundamental. Reaching answers, even tentatively, requires a safe environment. *The Unsupported Middle* certainly provided this 'still centre' with stimulation and also genuine unattributed sharing as formal designations were put aside and collaboration replaced the competitive and contracting mechanisms which have characterized the NHS internal market.

In December 1995 the format of *The Unsupported Middle* was deceptively simple. The five stakeholder groups, drawn largely from health authorities, community trusts, practice management, CHCs and non-executive board memberships, separately identified their aims and aspirations for a primary care-led NHS. They then split up into pairs and re-formed as new inter-stakeholder groups with representatives from the five 'home bases' in each. Their exploration and negotiation of each other's agenda then took up a full day, the second of the event. The NHS has a false familiarity – actually getting to know each other requires time, space and practice and in this case, expert external facilitation as well. Each of the inter-stakeholder groups had a 'professional outsider' in their membership.

What follows are the papers prepared by these five facilitators. They are not the stories of the individual groups as that would be quite wrong and of limited value now, even to those who took part. Rather, the following pages constitute the extension of some of the ideas, themes and images that began to form on the third day of the event, when the original stakeholder groups reviewed their learning and shared some initial thoughts and feelings in plenary sessions. By this time the critical issue was not power but interdependence. Personal growth had become as important a product as policy development. Common ground had been achieved in each group, and genuine empathy in some, when everybody honestly 'became a user'. The 'primary care-led NHS' slogan had been replaced by another strategy headline with its origins in Wessex – 'Achieving a Better Balance'. Above all, the opportunity which the reformed NHS gives us had been recognized and taken – to face 'the unsupported middle' which is in all of us. The rest of this book continues to address this subject. If a primary care-led NHS is really to succeed, it will need a new soundbite – for 'the unsupported middle' read 'the heart of the matter'.

Reference

1   Robinson R, Huntington J and Meads G (1995) *The Primary Care Challenge*. Churchill Livingstone, Edinburgh.

2 The people's champion?

June Huntington

Most general practitioners profess to be the patient's advocate. Consequently, it was disconcerting to discover that the users/CHC group feared a primary care-led NHS might place too much power in GP hands. In hospitals there are now managers who follow-up their patients' concerns or complaints about the care they have received from doctors. Having only recently secured this assurance, the group feared a primary care-led NHS would make it impossible in a general practice setting. Users already felt that the very structure of the practice – owned by the GPs and staffed by their employees – made it difficult to express concerns or to complain; while the number of practices in their districts and their 'independence' challenged CHCs' capacity to address issues in primary care.

Outpatient clinics in hospitals are increasingly organized by managers and 'staffed' by consultants and their associated medical and nursing colleagues. Similarly, inpatients increasingly receive communications from managers as well as doctors. These managers are not accountable to the doctors and can draw on the support of their own managers in following-up *with doctors* any concerns or complaints expressed by patients.

Many doctors in general practice, like those in hospitals, are courteous, kind and competent. They treat their patients neither as fools nor simply as bodies. But the concerns expressed by the users and CHC group remind us that the oft-quoted high levels of satisfaction with the general practitioner service, evidenced by many surveys, mask the negative experiences reported by middle-aged women, women with young children, and the elderly in other studies: concerns about access to the service, about the quality of attention and communication within the consultation, and about lack of respect and courtesy.

If managers have become the people's champion in hospitals, who is to take on this role in primary care? When the role of the potential new health authorities was first mooted, some commentators saw this essentially as that of 'the people's champion', using its strategic planning and purchasing power to bring health gain to local populations. Rapid development of GP fundholding and the difficulties of pulling resources out of the acute sector trimmed the aspirations of many health commissions even before they became health authorities in April 1996.

Some continue to take their people's champion role seriously, but acknowledge that to be recognized as such by local people they must be seen to ensure that users have a place, and more than this, an identifiable person or persons to whom they can take their concerns and complaints, in the knowledge that they will receive support in taking this up themselves or having it taken up on their behalf.

FHSAs differed in their performance of this role. Some continued in the tradition of the first Family Practitioner Committee administrator I ever met, who replied, when I asked if members of the public ever visited his difficult-to-find offices, that his was not a public complaints service. Other FHSAs chose to break the mould, taking more seriously their role as people's champion. Some of their staff who now work in the new health authorities are worried by the new primary care complaints system in which patients are expected to express their concerns of complaints initially *within the practice*.

Anyone who knows the full spectrum of general practice must feel that this change flies in the face of our knowledge of the way some GPs and their practice staff relate to their patients. The number of such practices may be small nationally, but some areas have more than their fair share. While some of these will have no practice manager, there is a risk that those who do will simply 'dump' the responsibility for establishing a practice-based complaints system on their managers, placing them at risk yet again of becoming an unsupported middle, not only between the patients and their GPs, but between the practice and the health authority.

This will not be a new experience for many practice managers who, alongside practice nurses, embedded the requirements of the 1990 contract into the daily life of the practice. They could not have achieved this without getting both GPs and patients on board. Many practice managers also played a similar role in embedding fundholding.

The guidance for general practices[1] makes clear that while 'local resolution' procedures at practice level should be 'practice owned', one person should be nominated to administer the procedure. It implies, though does not explicitly state, that the person will be an administrator; it also states clearly that 'if the person identified as practice complaints administrator is not a doctor, a nominated GP from within the practice should take a special interest in the operation of the procedure *and take ultimate responsibility for it'*.

GPs must heed this and not dump total responsibility on to their manager. Some GPs continue to be bitterly critical of the Patient's Charter, of which the new complaints system is an extension. If the practice manager is seen to embody the new procedure within the practice, there is a risk that GPs and other practice staff will project their hostility towards the scheme on to their manager. This risk is clear in the wording of paragraph 3.3 of the guidance for general practices document[1]: 'Everyone in the practice needs to sign up to the spirit of your practice-based system – all doctors working in the practice and all staff employed by the practice ... *no-one can be "above" the complaints system'* (italics mine). Paragraph 6.7, entitled 'Team Support', rightly emphasizes the need for any member of the team who is complained about to receive support from the person nominated to administer the practice procedure. The people management aspects of this task alone will challenge many practice managers, not least when a GP, or indeed, the practice nurse, is the focus of the complaint.

The guidance also recommends that practices engage in regular audit and review of complaints in order to learn from them: 'Regular review meetings would provide opportunities to discuss complaints received, consider identified training needs, and check that practice processes had been improved where necessary'. Some managers whose GPs continue to abhor any kind of practice meeting will find it difficult to engage them in this kind of learning.

The work involved in establishing and operating the scheme is considerable, so much so that practices are encouraged to keep a record of costs which can be used to support a bid for financial support from the health authority. What the guidance does not address is the psychological demands placed on any practice manager who undertakes this new role.

With the introduction of the Patient's Charter and the new complaints system into primary care, practice managers are increasingly undertaking what looks like a similar role to that of patient services and complaints managers in hospitals. The organizational context, however, is very different. While the GPs as 'directors' of the practice might allow and even encourage their manager to undertake this role, the manager who then advocates for the patient or mediates between the patient and the doctor will do so from the position of *employee.*

Those cast in the role of practice complaints administrator are recommended 'to approach your health authority's complaints manager' should they 'need help at any stage in setting up or running your procedure'.[1] But how will some GPs view their manager's seeking help from the health authority in such a delicate area of the practice's operations? Inevitably, if practice managers are given the role in most practices, they will forge ever closer links with health authorities, for those authorities have a duty to monitor the implementation of the scheme in practices and authorities.

In *The Primary Care Challenge* event, non-executive members of the new health authorities displayed considerable empathy with GPs, and with users and CHCs. Non-executives also tend to see themselves as 'people's champions'. They have important roles to play in mediating between users and providers of care, whether these be trusts or practices, whether on local strategic issues or in relation to complaints. They are perhaps even less likely than health authority managers to view GPs and their staff as proxies for patients. Unfortunately, their concerns as yet do not extend to practice managers, whose role within a primary care-led NHS is becoming increasingly critical as the focus of primary care provision shifts from 'the GP' to 'the practice'.

As that focus intensifies, practice management as a rapidly growing and changing occupation will attract increasing attention in ways that could bring discomfort both to individuals within the occupation and those who try to represent it. When the Association of Health Centre and Practice Administrators reviewed itself a few years ago, it chose to change its title to the Association of Managers in General Practice, not the Association of Managers in Primary Care. Since then, the Institute of Health Service Management has tried to attract practice managers towards greater identification with NHS management and managers.

The occupation, like that of its employers, is at a crossroads. Mirroring some of their employers, some practice managers are excited by the prospect of a primary care-led NHS, which offers them not only an extended role within the practice, but opportunities to work in trusts and health authorities as these occupations rush to develop their awareness of general practice and practice-based primary care. Some practice managers of today will lead the primary care organizations of tomorrow. Without serious development and support, others – like their GP employers – will remain confused and demoralized.

Practice manager participants in *The Primary Care Challenge* emphasized the need to involve the whole primary care team in developing a primary care-led NHS. Increasingly, practice managers are creating and sustaining conditions within the practice in which primary care team development can thrive. A report from a Scottish health education group survey of primary care teamwork in 11 Scottish practices found that team functioning had improved in the last few years.[2] They attributed this to 'the pro-active role of the practice manager as lynchpin and negotiator within the team which in most practices was a relatively new situation'.

The practice manager, in most practices, had been heavily involved in the decision-making processes in relation to the Health Promotion contract, and in some situations would take the lead by analysing the Health Board requirements and presenting them to the GPs for discussion. Their ongoing 'lynchpin' role for health promotion included managing the logistics of health promotion within the practice, coordinating relevant professionals, time-tabling rooms and clinic appointments, managing the collation of data, liaison with the Health Board, and deciding on, and securing, the necessary resources.

My own experience with many practices suggests that practice managers undertake a similar role in establishing and supporting new chronic disease management arrangements within the practice. The formerly rigid dividing line between clinical and organizational work is breaking down as clinical professionals increasingly take on board organizational aspects of their work, while non-clinical staff become increasingly involved in the organization of clinical work. We also know that many managers in fundholding practices are directly involved in specification, negotiation and monitoring their contracts with trusts.

Despite my having opened *The Primary Care Challenge* event with a brief discourse on power, and associated concepts of powerlessness, authority, influence, legitimacy and hegemony, participants seemed loath to discuss power. They discovered that others frequently perceived them as more powerful than they perceived themselves to be. Power also tended to be perceived in zero-sum terms – if one party got more, the other got less. Less apparent was any belief that new partnerships could be forged which would result in more power in the sense of greater potentiality to achieve improvement for service users – the unifying aim of all participants.

This should not be surprising when almost all groups felt like an 'unsupported middle' much of the time, not least the new health authorities, lying perilously between the NHS Executive and general practice locally. Charged with developing close working relationships (partnerships?) with GPs, they were also charged with 'monitoring' and 'developing' practices. As the people who increasingly embody 'the practice' as a corporate whole, practice managers will play more of a critical role in that emerging relationship as they do within the increasingly complex relational web of the practice itself.

Most practice managers, as both women and employees, will continue to exert *influence* rather than power, or will continue to say that this is what they do. The Shorter Oxford English Dictionary defines 'influence' as 'the exertion of action ... by one person upon another ... of which the operation is unseen except in its effects' or 'the capacity of producing effects by invisible means'. Some practice managers are leading, not just inside the practice, but beyond, in different kinds of interpractice groupings, and in the emerging relationship with health authorities. Sadly, some who have the competence and confidence to do this are being constrained by the parochialism and paranoia of their employers, and by the continued deference of their colleagues in other practices who prefer the role of organizational wife/mother/housekeeper to that of manager.

As practice managers at this event emphasized, however, existing limitations in their role and influence need to be recognized along with the essential nature and characteristics of general practice. Strategies for change are unlikely to be successful if they depend solely on practice managers as the agents for change within practices. Practice managers are often isolated from each other and from the wider environment. This must be addressed in practical ways, through secondments to heath authorities, use of practice managers as consultants, and promotion of mutual support and networking between managers themselves.

I have, in the past, urged health authorities to support the growth in occupational and organizational maturity of practice managers by consciously communicating with and relating to them.[3] I have since learned that such action may be perceived to breach the etiquette of employer–employee relationships. I remain convinced, however, that the new breed of practice managers can and must be able to make a wider contribution to the development of a primary care-led NHS. It is up to GPs and the new health authorities to enable them to do so.

References

1   NHS Executive (1996) *Practice-based Complaints Procedures: guidance for general practices.* Department of Health, London.

2   MacAskill S, Stead M and Eadie DR (1994) *Health promotion in primary care pilot.* Training project – initial interviews/final report. Centre for Social Marketing, University of Strathclyde, Glasgow.

3   Huntington J (1995) *Managing the Practice: whose business?* Radcliffe Medical Press, Oxford.

3 The Vicar of Dawlish holding the ring

Peter Key

The vicar was sitting by his altar preparing for a scheduled conversation with God. He was feeling uncomfortable. Twelve months ago he had wanted to reaffirm his flagging sense of mission. He felt he needed to focus his attention and energy, and had agreed with God that there were only two outcomes that really mattered:

1   did more people believe?
2   were more people living more worthy and compassionate lives as a result?

The idea was galvanizing; he set about his mission with new enthusiasm but quickly started bumping into realities which distracted and deflated him.

He was acutely aware of his own limitations and of the limitations of his resources. Could he really win over the doubters and cynics? He would look at his congregation from his pulpit – were they really on his side? Did they share his passion and conviction? Would they help in a practical way? And what about his fellow men of the cloth – he wasn't at all convinced that the Catholics and Methodists saw things in quite the same way as he did. There were even days when he suspected that they were really in competition with each other.

There were also the unavoidable distractions. It probably wouldn't increase the number of believers, but he simply must get the roof of the church fixed. And the delicate question of selecting a new choir master would have to be faced. Then there was the bishop. A good man who was kind and supportive but also a source of distraction at times. Was it *really* that important for him to be seen to address racial and ethnic issues in Dawlish? And what on earth could he do about the countless things which seemed to take his people from the chosen path and over which he had no control – from the National Lottery, to Sunday opening of supermarkets via soft porn on the television.

Reflecting on his situation, he decided that his conversation with God would be followed by a conversation with his good friend the chief executive of the health authority. They seem to share some common ground.

And what is that common ground? The opening session of *The Unsupported Middle* had seen a group of health authority chief executives construct a simple map of the power relationships within which they have to operate when pursuing goals such as a primary care-led NHS.

They had started by brainstorming a list of stakeholders with whom they had to work – and it was a very long list. Then they located those stakeholders within a map that had the appearance of a dartboard. Those stakeholders who were perceived to be powerful and influential would be placed around the bull's-eye. Those with little power and influence would be placed around the edge of the board. With a few notable exceptions (such as users), virtually all of the stakeholders occupied the bull's-eye!

It seems that a central dilemma for new health authorities (and for the Vicar of Dawlish) is that in pursuing worthwhile goals they are confronted with enormous complexity – diverging vested interests, limited internal resources and frequently having to operate through influence and persuasion rather than the exercise of control. In this context, the new health authorities' task of 'holding the ring', with so many stakeholders inside the ring, is at best daunting and at worst demoralizing. It can certainly lead to the feeling that the health authorities themselves could easily be another 'unsupported middle'. But, like the Vicar of Dawlish, theirs is a good and worthy cause which needs to be pursued with conviction and energy.

As the event unfolded and debate intensified, it became clear that there are some important and obvious messages that health authorities can draw upon that may help them make their vital contribution to the goal of a primary care-led NHS. These include the following.

The importance of leadership

New health authorities will need the wisdom of Socrates when addressing the population of Athens. They will need to inspire, and enthuse, and encourage, and win genuine commitment. They will need to demonstrate an enormous capacity for leadership, and not just from the top of the organization but throughout.

The message here is that the task of the new health authority is, in many ways, a specialized technical task which needs to be supported with real expertise from within. But that will never be enough because the task of 'holding the ring' demands leadership above all else and the style of that leadership will matter. Given the characteristics of many of the players inside the ring, an authoritarian approach will simply not work. Playing at 'I'm in charge' is unlikely to help because very often health authorities are not in charge of the events that will help to bring about a primary care-led NHS.

The importance of vision

It has become fashionable to claim that 'we don't know what a primary care-led NHS means' – profoundly unhelpful as a response. However, if this is not all posturing and there are real confusions, particularly at local level, about the future vision for the NHS, then the health authority in its informal leadership role will need to help all of the stakeholders answer questions such as: 'What is it we are trying to achieve through this policy initiative and what will it mean for me?'

The ever present danger is that efforts made to change the way in which health care is delivered will be openly or subconsciously resisted by stakeholders who have no vision of a preferred future, or no ownership of that vision. The danger will be magnified if the approach to change is then focused on systems and mechanics rather than on winning commitment to a new vision.

But what sort of vision? One of the dangers that was identified in the event is that the real purpose of the primary care-led NHS is seen as merely to shift power between different stakeholders. The danger with this perception is that it reinforces a view of the world in which the exercise of power and 'winning the game' is an end in itself. There is, of course, an alternative view which says that the world is a healthier place when power relationships are acknowledged as real but are exercised in relation to some common purpose and greater good which channels energy more constructively. It will arguably help health authorities enormously if they can ensure that the shared vision that they are helping to create is one of balanced and effective services where primary, secondary and tertiary care all play their part, rather than allowing the debate about the primary care-led NHS to degenerate into an unseemly power struggle.

The importance of collaboration

One of the powerful images that emerged from the event was of the NHS as an archipelago, with each island as an autonomous state. The waters between the islands were cruised by warships with guns primed. The message from the participants was of the need to scrap the warships and use the reclaimed metal to build bridges between the islands. The argument was that we must do so because there will not be any long-term winners if we do not. There may be some short-term gratification in winning the Battle of Jutland, but it will not last long if we know we cannot win the war. Above all else, we need to avoid the possibility of a pursuit of a 'primary care-led NHS' turning the NHS into another Bosnia, and the new health authorities have a major part to play in making sure that does not happen.

The bridges to be built by the health authorities will need to be both literal and metaphorical. The literal bridges will emerge from health authorities questioning how they communicate with the different stakeholders 'in the ring' and by what means. The metaphorical bridges will be built by health authorities looking for a style of working that can deliver long-term win situations rather than short-term gains won at a high price.

The importance of focus

The NHS has its equivalents of the leaking church roof, in abundance. One of the dangers facing the new health authorities as they pursue the goal of a primary care-led NHS is that their efforts and commitment will lead to little real progress, which in turn may result in rapid burnout and demoralization. If that is to be avoided, the new health authorities will need to be constantly challenging their own agendas in order to concentrate on those things that really matter, and constantly challenging their own ways of working in order to drive out those activities that do not work or contribute. It is easier said than done. It requires great self-confidence and self-discipline within the organization but the alternative is depressing both for those working in health authorities, and for those they are working for.

It goes without saying that the NHS Executive must play its part in helping the new health authorities to achieve this degree of focus. There seems to be a widespread consensus that the Executive is performing better than ever before in clarifying priorities and setting more realistic agendas, but that progress needs to be sustained and built upon if health authorities in turn are to be able to concentrate their attention and energies and make real progress.

The importance of patience

Rome was certainly not built in a day and perhaps we can never know how long it did take. We can, however, be reasonably confident that there were not many town planners around – neither were there any five year plans. Perhaps it was as simple as Romulus and Remus being right when they decided that 'this would be a good place to live' – and the rest followed. It is similar with the primary care-led NHS. This does seem to be 'a good place to live' but it is also a long-term vision that will not be fully realized for many years. But if that vision is clear and stakeholders feel committed to it, if we are always clear about next steps along the way, and if we have some small successes to celebrate, then there is a realistic hope that we will see genuine commitment to change and that new health authorities will feel a real sense of mission which will sustain them.

4 The death of Doctor Finlay? Trends and pressures in general practice

Peter Mumford

Introduction

The hypothesized 'unsupported middle' of the conference were practice managers and community services. As the conference proceeded my attention was drawn to general practice which began to look increasingly exposed and vulnerable as the sessions unfolded. Much emphasis has been placed on the new roles expected of GPs to create a primary care-led NHS; indeed, some see the future to be a 'GP-led NHS'. As the conference explored further the implications of these aspirations, deeply-felt concerns for the identity of general practice and the role of the GP emerged.

What follows is a collection of observations prompted by *The Unsupported Middle* conference. I am grateful to my colleagues at the King's Fund College, particularly Penny Newman and Gina Shakespeare, for their contributions to the ideas below, which came as we worked together on a new initiative for GPs.

Where next for general practice?

The 'primary care-led NHS' initiative places a new level of expectation on primary care professionals – that GPs, together with other community care providers, will take a more central role in providing and commissioning health care. This implies improving and extending the range of services they provide, and new and extensive collaboration with other professions and agencies, including commissioners, against a background of increased accountability and public scrutiny.

These expectations are being placed upon a service characterized by great variation in the range and quality of service it currently provides, and populated by practitioners, many of whom have chosen general practice to avoid having to work within the NHS bureaucracy. While some GPs welcome this new found responsibility and are actively engaged in this arena, many feel increasingly overwhelmed and disillusioned by the new demands and their impact on their role as GPs. Many feel frustrated and threatened by the undermining of their independence and increased external control of their practice. There is widespread low morale and poor recruitment to general practice. This is in strong contrast to the 1970s and 1980s when general practice developed a strong sense of identity, underpinned by professional development and the emergence of a number of individuals influential within and beyond the profession. The profession's success has been in establishing the distinctive and valued role of 'family doctor' in a changing health service, a role that now requires reassessment but whose grip on the profession threatens to block serious debate and analysis.

Trends and pressures

The conference highlighted a series of competing trends and pressures facing general practice. They include:

- The level of clinical work in general practice continues to rise. Patients expect more, know more and question more. The Patient's Charter imposes standards on general practice and the GP contract imposes tasks, some of which are considered by GPs to be of no clinical value. Complaints procedures are now explicit and have a higher profile. Together, these demands create more work and greater anxiety for many GPs. This is linked to the changing status of the profession in society and the fact that GPs' judgements are being questioned openly by patients. The result for many is a high level of additional stress.
- The primary care-led NHS offers GPs the opportunity to influence what needs to be done to improve the health of communities they serve. However, a tension arises between the need to identify and hold on to the 'core' of general practice and the desire to grasp the new agenda, with its attendant risks of being diverted from direct patient care. GPs working in the NHS are seen as central in implementing the changes associated with the primary care-led NHS and the signs are that they will come under increasing pressure, from commissioners in particular, to 'participate'.
- GPs have independent contractor status, but their well-being, income and the nature of their practice has always been dependent on NHS policy and practice. Accountability requirements are becoming more explicit and elaborate and are seen by GPs as increasingly controlling of clinical practice, and an additional administrative load. The current GP contract is seen by some GPs as a retrograde step, although to a large extent it is symptomatic of the current situation rather than the cause.
- Many of the current generation of GPs entering the profession (including a higher proportion of women) bring different expectations to the practice – shorter working weeks, out-of-hours cover, greater influence in the partnership early in their career, opportunities to undertake other duties to complement direct patient care and contemporary employment and management practices.
- Pressure to substitute nurse practitioners and other health professionals for GPs in some clinical (and managerial) roles is being welcomed by some and meeting strong resistance from other GPs concerned at the potential loss of the 'core'. Increasing incidence of direct referrals to other primary care providers is seen to undermine the supremacy of GPs as the primary gatekeepers.
- The rise of the specialist and the demise of the generalist in acute hospitals has highlighted the generalist role of the general practitioner, and raises questions over the nature and location of this role in the future. Sub-specialization in large group practices and across smaller practices is on the increase.
- Many GPs in their forties and early-fifties are weary of clinical practice alone and are looking for opportunities to undertake duties that they see to be complementing their clinical load.
- The partnership model is coming under increasing pressure. Practice management is becoming central to the future health of individual practices and is having an increasing influence on partners' clinical practice and challenging the traditional partnership model.
- Although it is unclear what a primary care-led NHS will look like, it is likely to accelerate the trend of extending the range of services provided by a larger primary health care team based around general practices, and include professionals from community and social services, presenting further challenges to the practice partnership.
- Similarly, the pressure for practices to collaborate in consortia arrangements (e.g. the out-of-hours co-operatives), multi-funds, total fundholding practice pilots etc., challenges the traditional partnership model.
- Recruitment and retention are seen in part as a symptom of the factors highlighted above and are currently precipitating further immediate pressures on practices and practitioners.

Outstanding questions and puzzles

These and other trends cannot just be taken at face value. The following questions lingered around the conference discussions:

- How real and sustained are the pressures outlined above? Which of them are part of abiding and long-term change, and which are passing fashion?
- What will emerge as the pre-eminent interpretations of the primary care-led NHS – indeed, what will be the next slogan as 'primary care-led NHS' fades?
- What spin will the main political parties find themselves putting on the NHS reforms in the lead up to the next general election?
- How far will the primary–secondary care balance alter in the face of rising pressures on acute services, particularly emergency services? Will the pendulum swing back?

Then there were the practical questions of implementation in general practice:

- What role will GPs sustain in commissioning?
- Is large-scale substitution of GPs' clinical activities possible or desirable? If so, what current GP activities could be dropped without eroding the 'core' role?
- What is the future for independent contractor status?
- Assuming the ideas behind the primary care-led NHS are pursued, will general practice develop the capacity, competency and understanding to contribute to commissioning, to bring about fundamental change in the organization of clinical practice, and to cope with its changing role?

Choices in general practice

The GP as an individual

The current trends and pressures on general practice are highlighting the choices facing GPs. Many are recognizing that they have to understand and actively engage with the NHS outside the familiar world of their own clinical practice. The choices as to where and how they contribute, beyond providing individual patient care, are opening up beyond the familiar roles of principal, GP advisor, clinical assistant, lead fundholder or involvement in medical politics. The new roles, particularly on the boundaries of organizations (general practice/commissioning, general practice/secondary care, inter-practice consortia etc.), may provide the basis for taking back some of the initiative, both personally and professionally, and create the potential for greater influence over improvements in the health of their patients and the local community.

The practice partnership

To 'step out' in this way presents risks for the individual and opportunity costs for the practice within which the individual is a partner. This tension has always been present but now takes on a new significance given the rising demands of patient care, and greater pressures on partners' time.

There have been recent and radical upheavals in general practice which have implications for the traditional partnership model, the most controversial and far-reaching of which has been fundholding and its derivatives. This has demanded new forms of leadership within and between practices and raised the profile, competence and authority of practice managers; in some cases creating multi-million pound enterprises with substantial sums locked up in new capital developments.

The trend is towards neighbouring practices discussing and doing 'business' together (where they may have remained isolated in the past), with or without the development of 'locality purchasing'. The choices now concern whether to consort with other practices in out-of-hours arrangements, sub-specialization, sharing of administrative services, etc. For some it is now a matter of 'how far and how fast'. Partners are becoming significant employers of practice staff, with the responsibilities of employment practice and management. Together these trends challenge the single autonomous practice model of general practice and raise questions as to the future for practice partnerships and independent contractor status.

Whither Dr Finlay?

Where does this leave the 'traditional' role of the family doctor? With the trend towards GPs spending more time away from day-to-day patient contact (continuing education, teaching, external clinical or management commitments etc.), the expectation of patients (à la Dr Finlay) that they can see 'their' doctor more or less any day of the week becomes untenable. This trend does not significantly threaten the 'family doctor' role from the patient's perspective although it may do so for the GP.

Of similar consequence from the patient's perspective is the increasing role of practice staff, particularly the nurse practitioner, in providing direct patient care. The GP's perspective on this typically falls into two camps – those who view this shift as an erosion of their core role and those who welcome the opportunity to share the clinical load.

The greatest challenge to the 'family doctor' role is wrapped up in the relationship between doctor and patient. It concerns trustworthiness: 'Am I convinced that "my" doctor is paying attention to my needs and using professional judgement to work out what is best for me, without letting other considerations, such as money, significantly sway his or her judgement?' This relationship lies at the heart of general practice and underpins the gatekeeper role and the success of primary care in the UK. If trust crumbles, and there are signs that it is beginning to, it will put immense new pressures on patients, GPs, commissioners and the whole system.

Conclusion

We cannot predict which of the above factors are going to have the most profound impact on general practice; indeed, there may well be more important factors to come which we have yet to see. However, the indications are that the changes that have been occurring over the last five years are just the beginning of a period of fundamental change in general practice that will continue through into the next century.

General practitioners play a central role in the NHS (90 per cent of patient contact happens outside hospitals, in general practice) and much is being expected of them in the development of the primary care-led NHS. GPs *are* part of the *'middle'* and they need all the support they can get.

5 A challenge from down under: comparisons between Australian and UK community and primary care services

Peter Mumford

In the closing session of *The Unsupported Middle* the facilitators were invited to offer personal observations. Much of the workshop had naturally looked at relationships and roles from within the health service, searching out and defining the 'unsupported middle', at times struggling to relate to the perspectives offered by 'users' participating in the workshop.

Our inclination in the workshop, when faced with the uncomfortable realities of being a user, was to slip from unquestioning deference to polite avoidance of what was being said. This belies the fact that we are all users of the service and testifies to the difficulties for health service staff in hearing what it is really like to be on the receiving end of their service. Users' perspectives can become intensely personal, challenge the true value of the service and expose the inappropriate emphases and limitations of new management arrangements and health policies, however worthy their aims.

The Unsupported Middle was held soon after I returned with my family from 12 months in Western Australia. One of my sons, Jack, now three years-old, was born with a chromosome disorder which has left him with severe disability. He's a great kid but can do little for himself and needs constant care and attention. My wife and I choose to have Jack based at home and seek practical support from health and social care services. We experienced a stark contrast between the attitudes of health and social care staff in Australia and the UK. In Australia we were asked: 'Tell us your needs and we will see what we can do', and 'This is our budget allocation for you – it's not much but how can we convert it into something of value to you?' There was a sense of possibility, of flexibility, of trying to understand our need and of adaption that we experienced within and between the social and health care agencies. The skills of the professional staff varied (as they do here in the UK), as did the relevance of particular assessments and therapies.

On our return to the UK we experienced a very telling contrast. We were frequently told: 'This is what we do here (you must fit your routine around us)', 'We will do an assessment (but there will be no choice of treatment **or** equipment when it is completed)', and 'This is what you need in your situation (we know what you need, you don't understand)'. In our estimation, the skills of staff, their commitment to their profession and to providing a good service were similar in the two countries – we have worked with some delightful people in both settings. However, the overriding impression we are left with, as carers here in the UK, is: 'Keep quiet and be grateful'. The net result is that the support we receive is less useful than it could be, and to receive it we have to fight through red tape, work out the Byzantine rules for ourselves, and be very determined, articulate and persistent. Of equal concern is that this leaves us, as carers, with little confidence in the service being able to adapt over time to even fairly modest change as Jack gets older.

Ours is not an isolated experience, nor are our needs particularly unusual for long-term carers. You can try and explain the contrast between Australia and the UK in terms of Australia being a 'new world' culture and the UK 'old world', or that money is the issue, but it does not lessen the starkly contrasted experience and outcome for us as carers.

Supporting carers is ideologically sound and an economic necessity for those working in primary and community care. Understanding the contrast described above between the Australian and UK experience, its causes and potential remedies, is critical for those of us who consider ourselves leaders in health care if we are not to project the mantle of 'the unsupported middle' out of the health service and on to the people we are employed to serve.

6 Delivering a primary care-led NHS

Eleanor Brown

By definition, a primary care-led NHS must start in primary care and, for many, this means general practice.

At *The Primary Care Challenge Part III, The Unsupported Middle*, representatives from primary care worked on their personal model of what the new primary care-led NHS would look like and in discussing this, identified areas which needed to be explored in order to move from the vision to the reality. Inherent in all the discussions was a feeling that everyone in the system could at any time feel like an 'unsupported middle', particularly in securing a firm infrastructure upon which to build the vision.

In the practical application of a primary care-led NHS there are unresolved issues. Perhaps the largest of these is whether partnership can remain as the foundation upon which primary health care is delivered. The current emphasis of corporate responsibility is evident in many of the recent changes within primary care. Accountability, new complaints systems, targets and needs assessment are all based on organizational achievements and responses and not upon individuals. This seems to be in direct opposition to the independent contractor status of the general practitioner and the somewhat old-fashioned concept of partnership, and appears as a halfway house between individual responsibility and a team approach.

The Concise Oxford English Dictionary describes 'partner' as 'sharer (with person or a thing); person associated with others in business of which he shares risks and profits'. The key words here are 'in business of which he shares risks and profits'. If we use this definition to describe general practice partnerships, then practice partnerships are based on the business of the practice in terms of financial risks and profits, leaving the health care aspect of the partnership to be dealt with by the general practitioner's individual contract with the Secretary of State through the rules and regulations of the *Red Book*.

At a time when society as a whole is questioning the partnership of marriage and many people are looking towards pre-nuptial agreements, perhaps it is time that general practice looked at their partnership arrangements and came to a more appropriate agreement for working within the recent legislation and which would sustain the movement towards a primary care-led NHS.

A partnership agreement may bind its partners to financial management of the business, but in terms of the delivery of health services, they may remain independent of one another and are not obliged to respond collectively. Recently, the Government has exploited this part of general practice partnerships to service their reforms. Fundholding has shown the way, bringing the partnership into the public domain through joint accountability for the fundholding budget, and setting the scene for further responsibility to be taken by the partnership rather than individually by each GP.

The concept of accountability provides a practical cue to a primary care-led NHS. The next step from financial accountability by the partnership is responsibility for quality and provision of services to patients by the partnership. At present, each GP has the ability to respond to any collective decision-making related to providing services for patients by acting within their individual contract. This individual accountability excludes GPs within the partnership acting as a true board of directors to set common standards of care which may be enforced through their professional and organizational structures. However, purchasing within fundholding is now not merely confined to services from outside providers. It is quite legitimate to purchase services from GPs with accredited qualifications for providing care within the fundholding scheme. This brings accountability into the arena of quality of care and services provided, and is monitored as such through the financial systems imposed and accreditation backed up by guidelines for care – almost a job description! But do existing practice business arrangements meet the new needs of this development in service delivery?

Partnership agreements do not usually make clear the role and responsibility of the general practitioner within the partnership. There is now much controversy with regard to how partnership agreements should be worded, with lawyers earning vast amounts of money to put together something which will stand up in a court of law. However, they still seem to be based on the ideas that, if someone is not adhering to the partnership agreement, it is up to the other partners to prove that the individual is outside the remit of the partnership document – difficult to do without having first established what partners' roles and responsibilities contain.

With the inevitability of increasingly complex primary care, it seems essential to outline clearly what is expected by individuals who deliver services. To date, the general practitioner is the only one within the primary health care team who does not hold such an outline in the form of a job description. But for how long is this acceptable, particularly when GPs' roles are developing and changing? Already we have seen much written on what the core of general practice is about. The idea that some practitioners will undertake core work whilst others undertake a mix of core and specialist services, and yet others may undertake a mixture of patient service provision and management of the organization, may lead partnerships to question the equity of workload within their organization, just as with many marriages. If a partnership document does not clearly set down anything but the financial arrangements it is hard to see how tension will not rise, and many more partnerships will feel the added stress of relationship breakdowns and the number of such partnerships will drop even further. Perhaps clarity of what is required of new practitioners would help raise recruitment into general practice.

In a world where contracts have become the norm and health authorities are beginning to look to contract with practices for care of populations over and above the immediate patients registered on their lists, partnerships need to look again at their own contractual relationship – the partnership agreement – and make sure that this is a robust foundation for delivering a primary care-led NHS.

7 Using the user

Kathryn Evans

It goes without saying
it goes without doing
(A health authority response to a user's question about making resources available to users)

I can understand the search for new terms to express changing relationships, however much I detest being a 'customer' on British Rail. So, I guess that 'user' is the best we can do. 'Patient', although I am happy to be a patient when I need to be, is undoubtedly passive and is associated with metaphors of illness rather than health. Also, I can never be a convincing 'client' unless I'm handing over guineas. So, as we gathered together for our exploration of 'the unsupported middle', we could all claim to be users of the NHS, BUPA subscriptions aside, and we could all claim to have some view of the experience associated with using services and how we would like it to be.

Use, however, is dependent on context, availability and differing needs. Even for those involved who were deemed to be representatives of users, and they were a small group, there were many complexities. Clearly, the CHC agenda was deemed different from that of user representatives and I had never thought before of how the interests of users and carers might be different too, especially in mental health and learning difficulty.

Representation is difficult, for once you become involved and learn about the system, it takes the edge off the naïvety that you may need to translate a fresh experience into insight. With the best will in the world you may be captured and made token, or collude with that from which you set out to remain independent. 'Using the user …'. Better perhaps to sweep up a group from the nearest shopping mall and hear from them as users.

The good intentions of everyone involved was not in doubt – this was clear from a résumé of all that the purchasers and providers in the group were keen to identify from their current practice. Managers routinely seek users' views. A good example may be the current listening exercise eliciting the views of all those, including users, involved in primary care, set in train by the NHS Executive. Whatever cynicism the Patient's Charter may provide, practices and trusts have conscientiously turned its requirements to good use. My experience of my GP practice and my local hospital outpatient department allows me to testify to that, and I have admiration for the organization of clinics, the orderliness of appointments, reduced waiting times and improved surroundings. Our group discussions cited other areas of improvement, for example in the quality and responsiveness of accident and emergency services.

Discussion identified too that as far as access to information is concerned, after a confused start, trust and health authority boards are trying to function differently and offer freer access to information for local communities. However, as an individual, information is only of use to me if I can make meaning of it. More may not be the answer. And, of course, what happens if, as a well-informed user, I end up demanding services or treatment that goes beyond budget or which challenges the wider interest. This is the stuff of newspaper campaigns. How easy in these circumstances to 'use the user' rather than venture to involve them, or to use the views that have been elicited. How do you hear, how do you ensure proper representation, how do you respond?

There was a realistic facing-up to some of the challenges underlying these questions. However much the statistics tell us about health and social care spending (£22.6 billion in 1978/79; £38.7 billion in 1995/96), what the users say and feel is that they experience decline. Where are the home helps? Rationing is a reality, a difficult notion to stand alongside choice. What about accountability at a local level? How are GPs to be held accountable? Where will the debate take place about resource allocation that will inform health authority decisions, and how?

Power was an explicit theme of the event and it surfaced in these issues and throughout. Often it was to reveal that one group attributed more power to another group than that group felt themselves to possess – but there were some realities. Everyone aspires to a more responsive service, so what stands in the way? That call for responsiveness is echoed again in the outcome of the listening exercise. 'Services should reflect the needs and preferences of the individuals using them. Patients should be able to exercise reasonable choice …'. To do so, they need comprehensive information about, and some involvement in, the services to be provided.

It is difficult to rebalance professional and user power. That is one of the realities touched upon again and again. An outstanding insight for me was that users saw managers as allies in asserting themselves in the face of professionals and carers. This is worthy of note in the current debate that surrounds the NHS 'bureaucrats'. NHS users tend to be deferential, disinclined to contest, challenge and confront. They get better and want to forget. Different groups want different things and could never agree. Besides, how can you realistically involve users in informed choices about their treatment? Who has been trained and paid to do what around here? Doctor knows best – never mind those few who become experts on their condition by reading it up via the Internet. This is despite the fact that many with chronic conditions know more about the totality of their experience across different facets of care than the professionals ever could. Professionals tend to overlook quality-of-life implications of their decisions, particularly for the elderly. They may hear but it may not influence what they do. How else do you explain the fate of evidence-based practice?

Again, however, the groups revealed their aspirations that things could be different. They felt managers had the scope to build real, not just token, involvement and ownership into their structures, with the possibility of influencing a culture of partnership between users and carers and providers and managers. But managers too need to be aware of what Chris Arguris calls 'professional incompetence'. NHS managers are an articulate bunch, adept politically, delivering good results, much of the time in the face of constant structural change. Their very skill, particularly in playing the game well and in dealing with structures and process, can become an obstacle to attending to the voice of the user.

Somewhere in all these discussions there are pointers for a way ahead. I joined the conference as one whose key experience of primary care has been as a user. In my innocence, I identified some potential.

The community health council – it exists, it has some statutory powers, it has some real talent in some of its officers. Why not review and rewrite its role? Certainly one of the purchasers in my group was keen to do so, only my facilitation skills got in the way!

Commissioners – the new authorities could move away from the fragmentation of services and find new ways of engaging users, in tailoring services to changing needs and offering options for treatment, in alliance with managers and professionals of course. Why not needs-led, outcome-driven purchasing?

Systems thinking – there is a growing awareness of the cost of fragmented services and a growing experience of new and user-friendly methodologies with which to energize networks, involve users and make connections across purchasers, providers, social services, voluntary organizations, businesses, environmentalists, through whole system events and their offshoots.

Citizens – where are you? Ultimately, that is what we all were – gathered in Bristol with a common interest in dialogue that can influence outcomes. Old habits die hard and I still tune into the *Observer* once in a while to catch Katharine Whitehorn, who is growing old gracefully and radically. She was acknowledging recently that empowering the patient is not as easy as it sounds and that when making long-term decisions about health, 'citizen' may be the only word to use – so I can sign off happily as a citizen.